THE JUICING FOR HEALTH RECIPES BOOK

A Beginners Guide to Juicing for Wellness

Nora C. White, RDN

Disclaimer

The information in this book is intended solely for informational and educational purposes. This book is not intended to provide medical advice and should not be used to diagnose or treat a medical problem

Copyright ©2023 Nora C. White, RDN

Table of Contents

The Juicing for Health Recipes Book

Nora C. White, RDN   5

Introduction

Juicing for health has become more and more well-liked over time. A concentrated beverage packed with vitamins, minerals, and antioxidants is created when the nutrients from fruits and vegetables are extracted. Juice and smoothie consumption has been linked to several health benefits, including increased energy, improved digestion, and weight loss.

One such is Anna, a 32-year-old mother of two who has had digestive issues and low energy for a long time. She experimented with a variety of diets and supplements, but her symptoms didn't get any better. She didn't start regularly juicing until she saw a significant shift in her health.

Anna began her day with a green drink composed of kale, cucumber, celery, lemon, and ginger. In addition to providing her with more energy, it helped her regulate her stomach. Fruit smoothies were her go-to snack throughout the day since they kept her satisfied until her next meal. Seasonal fruits and a variety of berries were used to make the smoothies.

After incorporating juicing into her routine for a few weeks, Anna noticed a significant change in herself. The stomach issues that had troubled her for so long were no longer a worry, and she had more energy than she had in years. She also noticed that her skin was brighter and clearer than it had been.

Anna's story is one illustration of how juicing for health may greatly enhance someone's wellness. Whether you're wanting to increase your energy, improve your digestion, or simply feel better in general, juices and smoothies may be a simple yet effective way to achieve your health goals.

The Juicing for Health Recipes Book

Nora C. White, RDN 9

Chapter One

Understanding Juicing

Definition of juicing

Squeezing, cutting, or mixing fruits and vegetables to extract the juice or liquid results in the process of juicing. The resulting juice may either be consumed on its own as a beverage or added to other foods. Vitamins, minerals, and antioxidants are often abundant in them. Juicing may include a wide variety of fruits and vegetables and can be done using a juicer, a blender, or merely by hand depending on personal choice and health goals.

Benefits of Juicing for Health

Juicing has several important health and fitness benefits. Some of the main reasons in favor of juicing include the following:

Increased nutrient consumption

Juicing makes fruits and vegetables more portable and easy to digest, allowing you to consume more of them. Juice made from fruits and vegetables often contains vitamins, minerals, and antioxidants that are essential for maintaining good health.

Improved digestion

The fiber in fruits and vegetables may be difficult for some people to digest. The body's capacity to absorb nutrients may be improved by eliminating some of the fiber from the juice.

Increased hydration

Many people struggle to drink enough water during the day, which may lead to dehydration and a variety of other health issues. Since that fruits and vegetables naturally contain a lot of water, juicing may help you keep more hydrated.

An increase in energy

A natural energy boost from the vitamins, minerals, and antioxidants in fresh juice may help you feel more alert and focused throughout the day.

Immune response boost

Fresh juice includes nutrients that may keep the immune system robust and protect the body from disease.

Detoxification

Juicing may help with overall wellness and health by getting rid of toxins and waste from the body.

Juicing is a fantastic way to increase your vitamin intake, improve digestion, boost energy, and support overall health and wellness.

Chapters Two

Various Juicers

Juicers come in many different kinds, each with unique features and benefits. The main subcategories of juicers are as follows:

Centrifugal juice

These sorts of juicers are the most common and often least priced. Fruits and vegetables are squeezed for juice using a fast-spinning blade. While being speedy and efficient, centrifugal juicers may not be the best choice for juicing fibrous foods like leafy greens.

Mouthheld Juicers

These appliances, sometimes referred to as slow juicers, squeeze and smash fruits and vegetables to release the juice from the food. They operate at lower speeds than centrifugal juicers, which could help preserve more of the juice's nutritious content. Masticating juicers are furthermore more efficient in juicing fibrous foods like leafy greens.

Citrus juicers

These juicers are designed specifically for juicing citrus fruits, such as oranges, lemons, and limes. The majority of the time, you push the fruit into a spinning motorized cone to extract the juice.

Juicers with two gears

These devices' two opposing rotating gears are used to extract juice from fruits and vegetables. While twin-gear juicers may be more expensive than other types of juicers, they are quite efficient and can produce a lot of juice from even the most challenging fruits.

Hydraulic presses for juicing

These juicers use hydraulic pressure to extract juice from vegetables, resulting in a highly concentrated, nutrient-dense drink. While preparing therapeutic juice blends or juice cleanses, they are often employed.

Integrated juicers

These juicers may be used manually and don't need electricity. They may also be used to juice other foods than citrus fruits, which is their typical purpose.

While choosing a juicer, take into account factors like price, ease of use, and the kind of vegetables you will be juicing. Even though certain juicers perform better with particular crop kinds, others may be more flexible. Your own needs and preferences will ultimately determine the best juicer for you.

Chapter Three

Juicing for Specific Health Conditions

Juicing is a popular and effective way to increase nutritional intake and encourage overall fitness and good health. Yet, did you know that juicing may also be tailored to address certain medical problems? Whether you want to improve digestion, reduce inflammation, or support a robust immune system, juicing may be a powerful tool for achieving your health goals. In this post, we'll discuss the benefits of juicing for a variety of medical conditions and provide suggestions and recipes for creating beverages that are specifically suited to your own health needs. Juicing may provide all-natural and effective support for a range of medical issues, from digestive issues to skin care.

Juicing for Weight Loss

Juicing is a great way to lose weight since it provides a nutrient-dense, low-calorie source of hydration that may help you feel full and satisfied. While juicing for weight reduction, it's crucial to keep the following strategies in mind:

Pay attention to veggies with fewer calories. When juicing for weight loss, it's essential to choose fruit that is high in nutrients and low in calories. Healthy alternatives include leafy greens, cucumbers, celery, and citrus fruits.

Employ a variety of produce

To ensure that you are ingesting a range of nutrients, it is crucial to mix and match different product types in your juices. Try combining leafy greens with cucumber and celery or citrus fruits with ginger and turmeric.

Avoid sugar-rich fruit

Even while adding fruits to your juice may be healthful, it's important to choose low-sugar varieties. Berries, apples, and grapefruit are all good options for fruits.

Take note of serving sizes

Although juicing may be a helpful addition to your weight loss strategy, it's important to pay attention to your portion sizes to prevent consuming too many calories. Try to drink one to two glasses of juice every day, and if needed, add in other balanced, healthy meals.

Provide a protein source and wholesome fats.

To help you feel satisfied and full, add sources of protein and healthy fats to your juices. Avocados, almonds, and seeds, as well as protein powder, are a few healthy substitutes.

Remain hydrated

Drinking water is essential for weight loss since it promotes healthy digestion and may be used to flush out toxins. Be sure you acquire enough water to drink during the day in addition to your juices.

By incorporating these tips and tactics into your daily juicing routine, you may create delicious, nutrient-rich juices that support your weight loss goals. Never start a new diet or fitness regimen without first talking to your doctor.

Detox with Green Juice

Ingredients:

Two celery stalks

A cucumber

One green apple

Lemon quarter (peeled)

A ginger root that is 1 inch long.

Method:

Rinse each component.

To put the apple, celery, and cucumber in your juicer, cut them into manageable pieces.

Start the juicer with all the items inside. Serve right away.

Strawberry-flavored Smoothie

Ingredients:

1 cup of berries, all kinds (strawberries, blueberries, raspberries)

Just one banana

Greek yogurt, half a cup

1 tablespoon of chia seeds.

Unsweetened almond milk in 1/2 cup

Method:

Cleaning is required in all areas.

In a blender, combine the mixed berries, banana, Greek yogurt, chia seeds, and almond milk.

After smoothing, blend. Serve right away.

Greens from the Tropics in a Smoothie

Ingredients:

A cup of pineapple, chopped

A half-cup of diced mango

A banana

A single serving of baby spinach

Unsweetened coconut milk in 1/2 cup

Method:

Mango and pineapple should first be cleaned before being cut into small pieces.

The spinach, pineapple, mango, banana, and coconut milk should all be combined in a food processor.

After smoothing, blend. Serve right away.

Carrot and Beet juice

1 little beet (peeled and chopped)

2 substantial carrots (peeled and chopped)

1/2 lemon (peeled)

A ginger root that is 1 inch long.

Method:

The beet and carrots must be washed,

peeled, and cut into small pieces.

Ginger, lemon, beet, and carrots must all be

included in a juicer.

Start the juicer with all the items inside.

Serve right away.

Smoothie with Almond Butter and Bananas:

Ingredients:

One banana

1 tablespoon of peanut butter.

One spoonful of sugar-free cocoa powder.

Unsweetened almond milk in 1/2 cup

1/2 a cup of ice

Method:

Chop the banana after peeling it.

A blender is used to combine a banana,

almond milk, peanut butter, cacao powder,

and ice.

After smoothing, blend.

Serve right away.

Enjoy these tasty and nutritious smoothie

and juice recipes if you're looking to lose

weight!

Juice from a Bowl of Slaw

Ingredients:

1/2 lb. that is green cabbage

14 pounds of peeled cloves of garlic

6 to 8 basil leaves

1/2 lb. with tomatoes

A pound and a half of green bell peppers

Method

Add the basil, garlic, and cabbage once the
tomatoes and bell peppers have been juiced.
Stir vigorously to combine.
Simply add everything to a blender and
puree until the mixture is perfectly smooth.

Salsa Spicy

Ingredients:

Green onions weighing 1 ½ pounds

A quarter pound of wheatgrass

1/4 pound of lemongrass

1/4 lb. fresh cilantro

1 lb. with tomatoes

1 lime

Method

When the green onions, wheatgrass, and lemongrass are processed in a juicer, the cilantro, tomatoes, and lime are added. Stir vigorously to combine.

Purée everything in a blender until it is smooth, being sure to peel the lime first.

Juice from Produce

Ingredients:

1/lb. of potatoes

Green onions weighing 1 ½ pounds

1 lb. with tomatoes

A pound and a half of green bell peppers

1/4 teaspoon of black pepper

Pinch of cayenne pepper

Method

Juice the potatoes, onions, and bell peppers first in a juicer before adding the tomatoes and bell peppers.

To combine the juice with the cayenne and black peppers, stir ferociously.

Simply add everything to a blender and puree until the mixture is perfectly smooth.

Picking Peppers

Ingredients:

½ jalapeno pepper

A pound and a half of green bell peppers

½ pound of cucumber

½ lb. with arugula

Method

Add the bell peppers and jalapenos to the cucumber and arugula juice thereafter. Stir vigorously to combine. Simply add everything to a blender and puree until the mixture is perfectly smooth.

Slim Juice

Ingredients:

4 basil leaves

Two garlic cloves

3 oregano leaves

1 green bell pepper

2 green onions

2 tomatoes

Method

Before incorporating the bell pepper, green onions, and tomatoes, combine the basil, garlic, and oregano in a juicer. Whisk vigorously to combine.

Margaritas Juice

Ingredients:

4 stalks of celery

Two apple

2 limes

Method

After juicing the celery, add the apples and limes. To blend, thoroughly stir.

Orange Juice

Ingredients:

Orange, one

1 lemon

One grapefruit

Method

In a juicer, blend all the ingredients by vigorously stirring.

Broad Sauce

Ingredients:

Celery stalks, two

3 tomato

Horseradish, grated, 1 teaspoon

½ lemon

½ lime

A quarter teaspoon of cayenne

Method

After juicing the lemon and lime, add the celery, tomatoes, and horseradish. Juice and cayenne pepper should be combined well.

Slim Energy Drink

Ingredients:

1 bunch of wheatgrass

½ inch of ginger

Sweet potato, half

½ lemon

Cranberries, 1/2 cup

Method

After juicing the sweet potato, lemon, and cranberries, add the wheatgrass and ginger. To blend, thoroughly stir.

A glass of Skinny Tea

Ingredients:

1/4 pound of peeled garlic cloves

Green bell peppers, 1/4 pound

6 leaves of basil

1 lb. of tomatoes

Method

In a juicer, blend the basil and tomatoes first, then the garlic and bell peppers. To blend, thoroughly stir. Just combine all the ingredients in a blender, then puree until completely smooth.

Digestive Health Juice

Juicing offers a concentrated dose of nutrients that may promote healthy digestion and assist to reduce digestive symptoms like bloating, constipation, and gas, making it a potent tool for enhancing digestive health. There are a few important tactics and ideas to bear in mind while juicing for digestive health:

Pay attention to products that are high in fiber: Fiber is a crucial ingredient for good digestion since it encourages regular bowel movements and prevents constipation. It's crucial to use food that is rich in fiber when juicing for digestive health, such as leafy greens, carrots, beets, and apples.

Employ herbs and spices that are gentle on the stomach.
Certain herbs and spices may reduce digestive inflammation and support a healthy digestive system. For their aid in digestion, consider using fennel, ginger, or turmeric in your juices.

Include foods high in probiotics
Probiotics are good microorganisms that may improve immune system function and

encourage a healthy digestive system.
Healthy gut flora may be supported by
adding probiotic-rich foods like kefir,
yogurt, or sauerkraut to your juices.

Keep hydrated

Digestive health must drink enough water
since it may keep stools smooth and aid with
constipation prevention. Together with your
juices, be sure you drink enough water
throughout the day.

Skip the sugary produce.

Although fruits may be a beneficial addition
to your juices, it's crucial to choose
low-sugar kinds to prevent aggravating
digestive symptoms like bloating or gas.
Berries, citrus fruits, and green apples are a
few nice choices.

You can make tasty, nutrient-dense juices that promote healthy digestion and aid to relieve digestive problems by adding these tricks and suggestions to your daily juicing regimen.

Pineapple Juice Mixed with Ginger

2 cups of chunky pineapple

A 1-inch long piece of ginger.

1/2 lemon (peeled)

Method:

Cut the pineapple into little pieces after washing it.

Peel and grate the ginger.

Add the pineapple, ginger, and lemon to a juicer.

With all the ingredients in the juicer, start it.

Serve immediately.

Carrot and Apple Juice

Ingredients:

3" long carrots (peeled and chopped)

2 green apples (cored and chopped)

A 1-inch long piece of ginger.

Method

It is necessary to wash, peel, and chop the carrots into little pieces.

Apples should be cut and cored.

Peel and grate the ginger.

In a juicer, add ginger, carrots, and apples.

With all the ingredients in the juicer, start it.

Serve immediately.

Mango and Papaya Smoothie

Ingredients:

1 mango (peeled and chopped)

Papaya, half (peeled and seeded)

A banana

Half a cup of Greek yogurt

1/2 cup of unsweetened almond milk

Method:

Cleaning and slicing into small pieces are required for mango and papaya.

Peel the banana and then chop it.

In a blender, combine the Greek yogurt, banana, papaya, mango, and almond milk.

Blend after smoothing.

Serve immediately.

Cucumber and Mint Juice

Ingredients:

Cucumbers, two

1/2 cup of fresh mint leaves

1/2 lemon (peeled)

Method:

Wash each component well.

Cut cucumbers into bits that will fit in your juicer.

Add the cucumber, mint, and lemon to a juicer.

With all the ingredients in the juicer, start it.

Serve immediately.

Kiwi and Spinach Smoothie

Ingredients:

2 kiwis (peeled and chopped)

One cup of baby spinach

A banana

1/2 cup of unsweetened almond milk

One tablespoon of honey

Method:

Kiwis need to be cleaned and sliced into very little pieces.

Blend the kiwis, spinach, banana, almond milk, and honey in a blender.

Blend after smoothing.

Serve immediately.

Beet and Apple Smoothie

Ingredients:

1 little beet (peeled and chopped)

Green apple one (cored and chopped)

1/2 lemon (peeled)

1/2 cup of unsweetened almond milk

One spoonful of honey

Method:

The beet has to be cleaned, peeled, and sliced into very small pieces.

Core and slice the apples.

Blender ingredients to be used are honey, almond milk, apple, beet, and lemon.

Blend after smoothing.

Serve immediately.

Watermelon and Mint Smoothie

2 cups of cubed watermelon

1/2 cup of fresh mint leaves

1/2 lemon (peeled)

1/2 cup of unsweetened coconut water

Method:

Wash each component well.

In a blender, combine the watermelon, mint, lemon, and coconut water.

Blend after smoothing.

Serve immediately.

Ginger and Turmeric Smoothie

Ingredients:

A 1-inch long piece of ginger.

Sliced into 1-inch pieces, turmeric

A cup of pineapple cut up into pieces.

1/2 cup of unsweetened almond milk

One spoonful of honey

Method:

Grate your ginger and your turmeric after washing them. Blend with almond milk, ginger, turmeric, and pineapple

Juicing to Enhance Immune System

Your immune system may be strengthened through juicing, which can also improve your general health and well-being. There are a few important practices and suggestions to remember while juicing to strengthen the immune system:

Concentrate on nutrient-dense produce: It's critical to choose produce that is high in essential vitamins and minerals like vitamin C, vitamin A, and zinc to promote immune system function. Leafy greens, citrus fruits, ginger, turmeric, and bell peppers are all healthy options.

Including immune-boosting herbs and spices: Certain herbs and spices may aid in immune system support and infection prevention. For the immune-boosting properties of garlic, Echinacea, or astragals, try adding them to your juices.

Including wholesome fats
Good fats, such as those in avocados and nuts, may aid in immune system support and inflammation reduction. To enhance your immune system, try using a handful of almonds or half an avocado in your juices.

Skip the additional sugars.
Excess sugar may worsen inflammation in the body and inhibit immune system activity. When juicing to strengthen the immune system, it's crucial to stay away

from added sugars and concentrate on full, nutrient-rich fruit.

Keep hydrated.
Water helps to flush out toxins and supports good immune system function, thus drinking lots of it is crucial for immune system health.

You may make tasty, nutrient-dense juices that boost immune system function and general health and well-being by adding these suggestions and methods to your juicing regimen.

Orange and Carrot Juice

Ingredients:

3" long carrots (peeled and chopped)

oranges two (peeled and chopped)

A 1-inch long piece of ginger.

Method:

It is necessary to wash, peel, and chop the carrots into little pieces.

Peel and dice the oranges

Peel and grate the ginger.

Oranges, carrots, and ginger should all be put into a juicer.

With all the ingredients in the juicer, start it.

Serve immediately.

Mango and Pineapple Smoothie

Ingredients: -

1 cup of chunky pineapple

1 cup of chunky mango

A banana

Half a cup of Greek yogurt

1/2 cup of unsweetened almond milk

Method:

Clean, and then chop up the mango and pineapple into small pieces.

Peel the banana and then chop it.

In a food processor, combine Greek yogurt, banana, mango, pineapple, and almond milk.

Blend after smoothing.

Serve immediately.

Berries and Beets

Ingredients:

1 little beet (peeled and chopped)

A cup of berries (strawberries, raspberries, blueberries)

A banana

1/2 cup of unsweetened almond milk

One spoonful of honey

Method:

The beet has to be cleaned, peeled, and sliced into very small pieces.

It is necessary to clean and chop the berries into little pieces.

Peel the banana and then chop it.

The beet, berries, banana, almond milk, and honey should all be combined in a blender.

Blend after smoothing.

Serve immediately.

Green Apple Juice with Spinach

Ingredients:

2 green apples (cored and chopped)

2 cups of baby spinach

Half a lemon, peeled (peeled)

Method:

Wash each component well.

Apples should be cut and cored.

Add the apples, spinach, and lemon to a juicer.

With all the ingredients in the juicer, start it.

Serve immediately.

Smoothie with Kale and Blueberries

Ingredients:

1 cup blueberries

Two cups of kale

A banana

1/2 cup of unsweetened almond milk

One spoonful of honey

Method:

Kale and blueberries need to be well-washed.

Peel the banana and then chop it.

The blueberries, kale, banana, almond milk, and honey should all be combined in a blender.

Blend after smoothing.

Serve immediately.

Turmeric with Ginger

Ingredients:

A 1-inch long piece of ginger.

Sliced into 1-inch pieces, turmeric

1/2 lemon (peeled)

Method:

Grate your ginger and your turmeric after washing them.

By squeezing it, squeeze some lemon juice into a little glass.

Add the ginger and turmeric to the glass.

Stir the mixture.

Have a drink now.

tomato juice mixed with bell pepper:

Ingredients:

2 large tomatoes

A red pepper (cored and chopped)

1/2 lemon (peeled)

Method:

It is necessary to wash and chop the tomatoes into little pieces.

After coring the bell pepper, chop it.

Add the tomatoes, bell pepper, and lemon to a juicer.

With all the ingredients in the juicer, start it.

Serve immediately.

Carrot and Ginger Juice

Ingredients:

3" long carrots (peeled and chopped)

A 1-inch long piece of ginger.

1/2 lemon (peeled)

Method:

It is necessary to wash, peel, and chop the carrots into little pieces.

Peel and grate the ginger.

By squeezing it, squeeze some lemon juice into a little glass.

The glass should be filled with ginger and carrots.

Stir the mixture.

Have a drink.

Mango and Coconut Smoothie

Ingredients:

1 cup of chunky mango

1/2 cup of unsweetened coconut milk

Half a cup of Greek yogurt

½ teaspoon of vanilla extract

One spoonful of honey

Method:

Clean, then chop the mangoes into very little pieces.

Blender ingredients include mango, coconut milk, Greek yogurt, vanilla bean paste, and honey.

Blend after smoothing.

Serve immediately.

Juicing for Healthy Skin

Juicing offers a concentrated dose of vitamins and minerals that may help to support healthy skin function and decrease inflammation, making it a terrific approach to enhancing the health of your skin. There are a few important practices and ideas to keep in mind while juicing for skin health:

Specify produce high in antioxidants. Antioxidants are crucial for maintaining healthy skin because they fight oxidative stress and soothe inflammation. Fruits and vegetables that are high in antioxidants include berries, leafy greens, carrots, and sweet potatoes.

Good Skin Nutrients

The proper function of the skin depends on several vitamins and minerals, such as zinc, vitamin C, and vitamin A. Bell peppers, pumpkin seeds, and citrus fruits are also good sources of these nutrients.

Including collagen-enhancing ingredients. Some nutrients may assist to increase the creation of collagen, a protein that is crucial for the health of the skin. Bone broth, kale, and spinach are all good sources of nutrients that support collagen.

Skip the additional sugars.
Avoiding added sugars and concentrating on full, nutrient-dense food is vital since much sugar may cause inflammation and breakouts.

Keep hydrated.

Water helps to keep skin moisturized and drain away pollutants, making it crucial for skin health.

You can make tasty, nutrient-dense juices that promote healthy skin function and minimize inflammation by adding these tricks and suggestions to our daily juicing regimen. As usual, it's crucial to speak with your doctor before beginning a new diet or exercise routine.

Potatoma Juice

Ingredients:

1 lb. of potatoes

6 leaves of basil

1 lb. of tomatoes

Method

In a juicer, first juice the tomatoes, then the potatoes and basil. To blend, thoroughly stir. Just combine all the ingredients in a blender, then puree until completely smooth.

Magic Skin Drink

Ingredients:

1/2 bundle of parsley

4 sprigs of mint

Alfalfa sprouts, 1 cup

One cucumber

½ lemon

Method

Juice the cucumber, lemon, mint, and sprouts before processing the parsley, mint, and sprouts. To blend, thoroughly stir.

Red Glow

Ingredients:

1 beet

1 pomegranate (or use 1 cup of cranberries as an alternative) 1 cup of chopped watermelon

Method

Juice the watermelon first, then add the pomegranate and beet after that. To blend, thoroughly stir.

Clear Potato Drink

Ingredients:

Four red or white potatoes

Method

In a juicer, process the potatoes.

Anti-Age Green Drink

Ingredients:

Spinach, 2 cups

1 head each of broccoli and cabbage

1 clove of garlic

Celery stalks, two

Method

After juicing the celery and garlic, add the spinach, cabbage, and broccoli. To blend, thoroughly stir.

Potato Melon

Ingredients:

1 sweet potato

1 potato, white

Cantaloupe, 1/4

1/2 cucumber

Juice the cantaloupe, cucumber, and potatoes in a juicer. To blend, thoroughly stir.

Envious Skin Drink

Ingredients:

1/4 lb. of broccoli florets

1/4 pound of cucumber

14 lb. of kale leaves

Green bell peppers, 1/4 pound

1/2 lb. of tomatoes

1/2 lb. of celery

Method

In a juicer, blend the broccoli, cucumber, and kale first, then the bell peppers, tomatoes, and celery. To blend, thoroughly stir. Just combine all the ingredients in a blender, then puree until completely smooth.

Beauty Juice

Ingredients:

1/2 pound of carrots

A half-pound cucumber

1/2 lb. of sweet potatoes

Carrot greens, 1/2 pound

1/4 lb. of arugula

Lemongrass, 1/4 pound

Method

Blend the carrots, sweet potatoes, and cucumber first, then add the carrot greens, arugula, and lemongrass. To blend, thoroughly stir. Just combine all the ingredients in a blender, then puree until completely smooth.

Green Juice

Ingredients:

Two stalks of celery and one cucumber

1 apple

1 cup of spinach

1/2 lemon (peeled)

A 1-inch long piece of ginger.

Method

Well-wash each part of the green goddess juice.

Cut the apple, celery, and cucumber into manageable pieces to put in your juicer.

With all the ingredients in the juicer, start it. Serve immediately.

Berry Smoothie Explosion

Ingredients:

1 cup of berries, all kinds (strawberries, blueberries, raspberries)

A banana

Half a cup of Greek yogurt

One spoonful of honey

Half a cup of almond milk

Method

Clean every component.

The mixed berries, banana, Greek yogurt, honey, and almond milk should all be combined in a blender.

Blend after smoothing.

Serve immediately.

Pineapple and Kale

Ingredients:

1 cup of kale that has been finely chopped

A cup of pineapple cut up into bits.

A banana

1/2 cup of unsweetened almond milk

1/8 teaspoon grated ginger root

One spoonful of honey

Method

Before producing a smoothie, the kale and pineapple need to be rinsed and chopped into little pieces.

Blend the kale, pineapple, banana, almond milk, ginger, and honey in a blender.

Blend after smoothing.

Serve immediately.

Enjoy!

Juicing for Detoxification

Juicing can be a helpful tool for liver health promotion and body detoxification. The liver is in charge of removing waste products and poisons from the body, and some nutrients may promote this process. There are a few important techniques and tips to keep in mind when juicing for detoxification:

focus on foods that help the liver Detoxification and healthy liver function can both be supported by some foods. Leafy greens, cruciferous veggies, beets, and citrus fruits are also healthy options.

Include cleansing nutrients. The liver's detoxification activities may be supported by certain nutrients, such as glutathione, selenium, and B vitamins. Mushrooms, nuts & seeds, and leafy greens are all good sources of these nutrients.

Use bitter greens.

Dandelion and arugula greens, which are both bitter, may encourage bile flow and promote good liver function.

Take in a lot of water.

Water consumption is crucial for flushing toxins from the body and supporting healthy digestion.

Skip the additional sugars.

Avoiding added sugars and putting your attention on the whole, nutrient-dense produce is important because excess sugar can cause inflammation and interfere with healthy liver function.

You can make delicious, nutrient-dense juices that support healthy liver function and encourage detoxification by incorporating these suggestions and methods into your juicing routine.

Detox with Green Juice

Ingredients:

2 green apples (cored and chopped)

A cucumber (peeled and chopped)

Four celery stems

1/2 lemon (peeled)

A 1-inch long piece of ginger.

Parsley garnish

Method:

Wash and chop each into small pieces for each ingredient.

All ingredients are placed in the juicer.

With all the ingredients in the juicer, start it.

Serve immediately.

Beverage for Beet Detox

Two enormous beets (peeled and chopped)

Două carrots (peeled and chopped)

A 1-inch long piece of ginger.

1/2 lemon (peeled)

Method:

Washing and chopping into small pieces are required for beets and carrots.

Peel and grate the ginger.

By squeezing it, squeeze some lemon juice into a little glass.

Add the ginger, carrots, and beets to the glass.

Stir the mixture.

Have a drink now.

Blueberry Detox Smoothie

1 cup blueberries

A banana

Half a cup of Greek yogurt

1/2 cup of unsweetened almond milk

1 tablespoon chia seeds

Method:

Cleaning blueberries is necessary.

Peel the banana and then chop it.

The blueberries, bananas, Greek yogurt, almond milk, and chia seeds should all be combined in a blender.

Blend after smoothing.

Serve immediately.

Turmeric Juice

1 little beet (peeled and chopped)

Două carrots (peeled and chopped)

A 1-inch long piece of ginger.

Sliced into 1-inch pieces, turmeric

1/2 lemon (peeled)

Method:

Washing and chopping into small pieces are required for beets and carrots.

Peeling and grating ginger and turmeric are required.

By squeezing it, squeeze some lemon juice into a little glass.

Add the beets, carrots, ginger, and turmeric to the glass.

Stir the mixture.

Have a drink now.

Spinach Detox Smoothie

Baby spinach, 2 cups

A banana

Half a cup of Greek yogurt

1/2 cup of unsweetened almond milk

One spoonful of honey

Method:

Baby spinach should be cleaned.

Peel the banana and then chop it.

In a blender, mix the baby spinach, banana,

Greek yogurt, almond milk, and honey.

Blend after smoothing.

Serve immediately.

Orange and Carrot Detox Juice

4 large carrots (peeled and chopped)

Oranges two (peeled and chopped)

A 1-inch long piece of ginger.

Method:

It is necessary to wash, peel, and chop the carrots into little pieces.

Peeling and dicing oranges is a good idea.

Peel and grate the ginger.

Ginger, oranges, and carrots should all be put in a juicer.

With all the ingredients in the juicer, start it.

Serve immediately.

Lemon and Cucumber Detox Drink

A cucumber (sliced)

1 lemon (sliced)

1 liter of water

Method:

Slices of lemon and cucumber should be cleaned.

The cucumber and lemon should be poured into a large pitcher.

Add water to the pitcher.

Stir the mixture.

Place in the refrigerator for at least one hour before serving.

Detox Smoothie with Pineapples

1 cup of chunky pineapple

A banana

1/2 cup of unsweetened coconut water

Half a cup of Greek yogurt

A little bit of kale

Method:

Spotless pineapple slices

Peel the banana and then chop it.

Clean the kale.

Kale, pineapple, banana, Greek yogurt, and

coconut water are all blended.

Blend after smoothing.

Serve immediately.

Apple and Ginger Detox Juice

2 green apples (cored and chopped)

A 1-inch long piece of ginger.

Several mint leaves

1/2 lemon (peeled)

Method:

Clean, then slice the apples into small

pieces.

Peel and grate the ginger.

Mint leaves need to be trimmed and cleaned.

By squeezing it, squeeze some lemon juice into a little glass.

Apples, ginger, and mint leaves should all be poured into the glass.

Stir the mixture.

Have a drink now.

Detox Smoothie with Watermelon

2 cups of pieces of watermelon

1/2 cup of unsweetened coconut water

Half a cup of Greek yogurt

One spoonful of honey

Method:

After washing, the watermelon should be sliced into little pieces.

The watermelon, coconut water, Greek yogurt, and honey should all be combined in a blender.

Blend after smoothing.

Serve immediately.

Detox with Apple Juice

Ingredients:

Two pounds of green apples

1.2 lbs. of mint leaves

1 lemon

Orange, 1

One cucumber

Method

Juice the apples, mint, lemon, orange, and cucumber in a juicer before adding the other ingredients.

To blend, thoroughly stir. Just combine all the ingredients in a blender (be careful to peel the orange and lemon first!) and purée until completely smooth.

Kale Juice

Ingredients:

1/2 pound of mustard greens

1/2 lb. of kale leaves

1/4 lb. of parsley

1 lb. cucumber

1/2 lb. of celery

Method

After juicing the cucumber and celery, add

the dandelion greens, kale, and parsley.

To blend, thoroughly stir.

Just combine all the ingredients in a blender,

then puree until completely smooth.

Fennel Cleanse

Ingredients:

1/4 pound of peeled garlic cloves

1/2 lb. fennel

1/2 lb. of kale leaves

8 leaves of basil

Two pounds of tomatoes

1/4-pound cucumber

1 lemon

Method

The tomatoes, cucumber, and lemon are processed in a juicer after the garlic, fennel, kale, and basil. To blend, thoroughly stir. Just combine all the ingredients in a blender (be careful to peel the lemon first!) and purée until completely smooth.

Green Diet Drink

Ingredients:

Green bell peppers, 12 pound

1/4 lb. of broccoli florets

1/2 lb. cucumber

1/2 lb. of cabbage

Method

In a juicer, first juice the bell peppers and broccoli, then the cucumber and cabbage.

To blend, thoroughly stir.

Just combine all the ingredients in a blender, then puree until completely smooth.

The Purifier

Ingredients:

1 lb. of spinach

1 lemon

1/4 lb. of parsley

1/2 lb. of celery

Method

After juicing the celery and parsley, add the spinach and lemon.

To blend, thoroughly stir.

Just combine all the ingredients in a blender (be careful to peel the lemon first!) and purée until completely smooth.

Chapter Four
Juicing Tips and Techniques

Some various strategies and practices may help you get the most out of your juicing experience, whether you are new to juicing or trying to enhance your juicing abilities. Here are some crucial juicing pointers to remember:

Choose the proper food: When choosing produce for juicing, it's crucial to pick out fresh, high-quality fruits and vegetables that are free of imperfections or decay indications. Although toxic pesticides and other chemicals are less likely to be present in organic vegetables, it is also a wise option.

Produce should be well washed before juicing to eliminate any pathogens or dirt. If you're using non-organic vegetables, this is very crucial.

Produce preparation: Be careful to chop your produce into tiny, manageable pieces so that your juicer can handle it. Although tougher food like apples or carrots may be sliced into smaller pieces, leafy greens should be tightly wrapped and carefully fed into the juicer.

Rotate between soft and firm vegetables while juicing to avoid clogging and guarantee a constant, smooth flow of juice.

This may assist in keeping the juicer operating efficiently and avoiding clogs.

Combine flavors: Play around with various flavor pairings to discover your favorite juice creations. To boost the taste and nutritional value of your juice, you may also add herbs or spices like parsley, ginger, or turmeric.

Drink your juice right away: Juice should be taken as soon as it is created since it loses taste and nutrients over time. If you must preserve your juice, be sure to do it in a refrigerated airtight container and use it within a day.

You may make scrumptious, nutrient-dense juices that help you achieve your health and wellness objectives by using the juicing strategies and procedures described here. Juicing may be a useful tool for attaining your health objectives, whether you want to enhance digestion, lessen inflammation, or strengthen your immune system.

Chapter Five
Conclusion

Congratulations! Your amazing trip into the realm of juicing for health has just come to an end. We have discussed the various advantages of drinking fresh juices throughout this book, including better digestion, greater energy, radiant skin, and others.

We hope that this book has given you the information and motivation you need to advance your health and fitness, whether you're new to juicing or a seasoned veteran. From the many kinds of juicers to the significance of utilizing high-quality products, from the essential nutrients included in various fruits and vegetables to the numerous health advantages of juicing, we have covered a broad variety of issues.

Above all, we want you to start juicing for yourself after reading this book. Juicing is an effective method for enhancing your health and wellness because of its wealth of health advantages and mouthwatering tastes. Fresh juices may help you reach your objectives, whether you want to reduce weight, improve digestion, or just feel more energized.

So why are you still waiting? Start experimenting with various fruits and veggies in your juicer by grabbing them.

You may make tasty and nourishing juices that will aid you in achieving your health and wellness objectives by using the advice and methods in this book. And keep in mind that juicing is just one aspect of a healthy lifestyle. Therefore, be sure to combine your juicing regimen with a healthy diet, consistent exercise, and plenty of downtimes.

We appreciate you coming along with us as we explore the world of juicing for wellness. We wish you success as you work toward bettering your health and wellness!